I0787491

Brain Injury - From This Guy's Perspective

TBI - What You Can't See

by

Joseph Brewer

Brain Injury - From This Guy's Perspective

TBI - What You Can't See

Printed in the United States of America.

First Printing, 2021

akaJoeBrewer.com
Psalm 84:10

TABLE OF CONTENTS

Introduction 1

Chapter 1 - What You Can't See 5

Chapter 2 - Additional Discoveries and Understandings 17

Chapter 3 - Redundancy and Hypersensitivity 23

Chapter 4 - Friends 29

Chapter 5 - My Thoughts on Depression 37

Introduction

So you can grasp what life is like for your friend or loved one who lives with a Traumatic Brain Injury (TBI), I will grant you a look into my world, post-injury. Since I'm a 57-year-old guy, this will be from my perspective. I have moved beyond some of these things, by the grace of God. However, after interacting with fellow TBI survivors for a few months, I found that most of the items I list below are commonplace for all (TBI) survivors. Finding out that others go through the same things as you do is comforting, although alarming, because you don't wish this on others, and you realize that it really did happen to you. You can no longer dismiss it; it happened to you.

I'm 18 years post-injury. For the first few years, no one knew I had a TBI. All we knew was my body had changed. Weird and bizarre things were happening I could not understand. Things like numbness from my face to my waist on the left side, left eye watering so bad it was like someone turned on a faucet, chronic fatigue, cramping on the left side, pressure in my head, inability to handle loud sounds, the flashing of lights causing nausea, confusion, fatigue, shooting pains in my head, overwhelmed by simple tasks, loss of smell and taste, and so on. On the left side of my head, there appeared to be signs of the electricity's path where my hair was turned backward and, at the end of that line of hair, there was a spot that caused debilitating head pain if pressed on.

I had 240 volts or 480 volts of electricity enter

my left forearm and exit both sides of my head. I was told I blew a puff of smoke from my mouth. I'm guessing it was from the metal fillings in my teeth liquefying as the electricity passed through them. I had to have the fillings replaced three months later.

For some added context, before my TBI, I worked 24 years of industrial construction (welding, mechanical, piping, rigging, operating equipment, and so on), with the last 15 years as a foreman. I was in 2 automobile accidents where the vehicles I was in were both totaled. I rolled my truck several times on the freeway, and in the other accident, I was rear-ended with such an impact it buckled the frame of my car. I also had 2 earlier industrial injuries requiring surgery, ligament reconstruction on my right ankle, and arthroscopic surgery on my right knee. In all of these, however, I'm of the opinion that it was God's means of preparing me to mentally and emotionally survive my brain injury. God also proved He would provide for me and my family.

My latest diagnosis is that my brain functions like I have a concussion with PTSD and often stuck in fight-or-flight mode. I'm hypersensitive to light and sound. Although I am not experiencing the mental and emotional effects of depression, my body responds to my brain injury as though I am depressed, so it is dumping cortisol on an endless cycle.

Chapter 1 - What You Can't See

The following are my experiences over the past 18 years. Your TBI survivor has likely gone through or is going through some similar experiences, too.

- They may be in a state of complete sensory overload where their entire focus is on not panicking or blacking out from it. And they didn't even see it coming. All they did was make their way through a crowd, and the movements set it off, or the sounds surrounding them blended into a symphony of screeching sounds in their head.

- They may be overwhelmed by the sounds of their current environment. Percussive sounds feel like a rubber mallet being bounced off their brain. High-pitched sounds feel like a siren has been played in their head. Indistinct chatter or multiple conversations surrounding them creates sensory overload.

- They may be so fatigued that they can barely speak words today. It's likely because they were around people yesterday that demanded their attention.

- They may have a giant void in their vocabulary today that wasn't there yesterday. It's like 3/4 of their vocabulary was just deleted from their brain, so thinking is a challenge, and communication may not be possible at that moment. The words aren't even on the tip of their tongue because they are just gone. Stuttering like a fool is the rule of the day. They are likely wondering if it is a permanent condition this time. Statistically they know it should not be due to all the previous episodes, but they are so broken today they cannot process that.

- They likely go through moments, in the day, of fear they have to control and calm. When their brain seems to shut down and quits functioning normally, it creates those moments of fear.

- They wonder if they are acting weird because they can't tell but know their brain has a glitch at the moment. Their eye movements flit around. They are likely self-conscious and somewhat embarrassed at this moment but trying to conceal it from you, which makes it worse. They don't want you to become uncomfortable being around them.

- They may look like they are listening to you and even nodding their head, but their brain can't keep up with you today or even process the words you're saying. They feel bad because they want to but don't know how to tell you. They're also afraid you will just avoid talking to them if they tell you.

- They wonder if their condition will get worse than it is at present because they have such low brain function at times.

- They are worried that they are just letting everyone they love down because they can't assess their participation in life.

- They are trying hard not to feel sorry for themselves today, but that requires what seems like an incredible mental and emotional effort, sometimes. They may not have that ability at this moment but would surely get over it.

- They feel somewhat isolated in their brain because of the uncertainty of how their brain functions. They can't tell if their words and actions are making sense. The level of frustration this creates is incredible.

- They may have just walked through the house looking for the fire that their brain tells them is there from the phantom smells. They may touch walls looking for an abnormal heat source.

- They try to stay positive, but sometimes, that is an overwhelming chore.

- That they showed up at all tells you how very important you are to them or how important the event is. It took all they had just to be there today. They probably did nothing the last couple of days so they could be there with you.

- They can't read today. The words are all jumbled up and make no sense. They can read today but can't process the message conveyed.

- They canceled all their plans for the day at a moment's notice because they do not have the ability to participate in life today. Sorry for the inconvenience. The disappointment their family goes through because of it weighs on them.

- They see those who are skeptical of their injury because they can't see the damage in their head, and on the outside, they look normal. So, now, they are dealing with being thought of as fraud and a liar. Thanks for that!

- What seems simple to you may overwhelm them, but they try to hide it so they can take part in life with you.

- You know those little things you do like sleeping, breathing, and swallowing, yeah, well, those have frequently been a challenge for them. There are times when they actually have to work at breathing and swallowing because it's like their brain simply forgot how to do them. Sleep has become a less than productive time in their life. They sleep, but if they reach REM sleep, then it's like they ran a marathon while sleeping, so they are in worse shape than before sleeping. Daily naps are required to maintain a pleasant disposition and maintain life.

- They may have pain in multiple areas of their head and for an undetermined amount of time. While they used to eat pain like candy, now, even the smallest pain excites their brain and is like a flashing beacon screaming, I hurt, I hurt, I hurt!

- They may lack empathy or, at least, appear to lack empathy. It's not that they don't care. It's just that their daily battles take so much from them that, sometimes, there isn't anything left for anyone else. This also weighs on them. It may also be a processing issue. They are not certain if they're reading your situation correctly.

- They remember what they used to do but can no longer perform at that level. It's difficult for them to take. Sometimes, they feel less a man because of it.

- They get very frustrated because they have many projects to work on but have to choose between cleaning up from the last project or starting this next project. They had enough physical stamina and mental energy to get the last project done but not the cleanup part of the program.

- Light may be too much for them today. Light may cause them tremendous stress today. Their brain just can't handle it, and they don't know why.

- Sorry, but no, you don't know how they feel just because you're getting old. They're getting older also and recognizes the difference. You do realize that after a fashion, you're calling them a liar, right?

- You really do not understand what you're asking when you ask them to be social. Being social requires planning, days of planning. Asking them to be social means asking them to give up several days of their life so they can rest up before your social event and then spend days recovering following the event. Although you do not realize it, you're asking them for a week of their life to be part of your social life. Please, value the time you have with them, since they may very well have given you a week of their life in the few hours you had together.

- They used to drive for hours on end, but now

10 minutes may be a challenge, and the focus it takes is a fatigue multiplier.

- Putting pen to paper used to be as simple as breathing. Today, just signing their name multiple times like on a real estate contract will cost them 12-24 hours of their life trying to recover from it. Whatever the process it is that creates and conveys information from their hand to paper, it no longer functions like it used to.

- It may seem silly, but fidgeting seems to promote focus. Distracting their body with small movements seems to make it easier to focus on the task at hand, including listening to someone talking.

- Claustrophobia has taken on a whole new meaning. It used to only be in confined spaces or restraint, but today, it comes from being in a crowd, stuck in the middle of a row with people all around them, or even the inability to remove themself from the sounds of the crowd. Even just bumping into something may bring it on. It can also create an instant rage that they have to overcome.

- They used to attend movies at the theater, but today, the movement on the screen causes them something akin to a seizure. The better the picture quality, the worse their reaction to it. The newer 4k televisions seem to have the same effect due to their depth of field.

- To avoid becoming agitated, they have to avoid places that will make them yell, speak in elevated tones to communicate or speak over other sounds. Something about them having to maintain a loud tone provokes them. They do not understand why this happens, but it does.

- When they tell you about their life and what

they go through, it's not for your pity and sympathy. It's so you understand. It's so you understand when they say they can't talk right now or go with you right now because their brain is broken. It's so you understand when they have to cancel on you or just tell you no. And, it's because you matter to them, and they deeply care for you.

Chapter 2 - Additional Discoveries and Understandings
March 2019 Update

- Their brain injury does not mean they suffer from a loss of intellect or common sense. When their vocabulary disappears, they will have difficulties drawing upon their intellect. We think in the form of words, so when they disappear, there are no resources to draw from. It's not the intellect that has declined; it's the ability to draw from it as a resource that is impaired today.

- Their dreams have occasionally become strange in that they are like rapid flashes of images rather than that feeling of experiencing the moment. After several of these rapid flashes, they may have to get up from bed to clear their head and stop this cycle of dreaming.

- It takes significantly longer for them to make a habit change now than prior to their injury. Breaking an old or forming a new habit is, at minimum, a 6-month proposition to even begin making this change of habit. This can be hard for them to take. They know they want to make a change, but it is just going to take time. And no, reminders do not work for them. Because of their brain function level at the time of the reminder, they may or may not even be able to consider it. Just the reminder popping up and their inability to complete the task can weigh heavily on them. For them, it's another in a series of what feels like failures.

- Naps have now taken a weird turn for them. When they say they have to sleep in the middle of the day, it is because they are experiencing what feels like a complete system failure. It feels like their brain and body are shutting down. It's like, suddenly, their life force is leaving their body, and if they do not sleep, they may not survive the day. You know how when your phone or laptop battery is used up, all the bars are empty, it turns from green to red and has that red slash mark through the battery where you know it is just going to shut off at any moment. That's kind of what it feels like, only it's their lives we're talking about here.

- They may seem disinterested while on something like a road trip, but that is not the case. The constant changes in scenery, food, places to sit, sleep, shop create sensory overload. In their element (home), they have their life ordered so they can function in it as close to a normal existence as possible. Out there on the road, that is not possible. Most of the time, their mind will be blank from dealing with almost constant sensory overload and being pushed out of their element. Whether you or they realize it, at home they have arranged their normal day-to-day environment in a way that allows them to adapt to their ever-changing life. This becomes obvious as travel strips them of all their built-in securities that make their life feel somewhat normal.

- Playing with their phone while you drive is likely to minimize sensory overload. In wide open spaces where the movements are slower due to being further away they may not need the stability of focusing on their phone.

- Seriously, you do not understand just how much they miss working. As they drive past places they might have worked or see people performing tasks they used to do, they may become somewhat depressed. It truly is discouraging seeing others working in their previous profession when they know they can no longer function in that capacity. It's something of a kick to the gut for them. In that moment, it strips them of their manhood, reminds them of their loss, and takes them to a dark place, inside, that they try to avoid.

- Apologies in advance for the anger and outrage shown in this paragraph, but if you have read the earlier version of this essay and still have the audacity to say to them, "you get to stay home tomorrow" or "at least you don't have to work tomorrow", you really must be a selfish and pathetic person. For you to say something like that to them, you must be a very sad and small person inside who, in reality, only ever thinks of yourself. It's bad enough to think it, but to say it to them? Your envy, bitterness, and pettiness must really drag you down deep. Your very existence must be miserable. You know, even with all they are going through, it's likely that they almost feel sorry for you having to survive such a miserable existence created by your own hand.

Chapter 3 - Redundancy and Hypersensitivity
February 2021 Update

This update feels like it's about redundancy and hypersensitivity.

I have never liked the city. It's always felt somewhat claustrophobic for me, but it has gotten far worse since my last update. I constantly feel as though I need to run away to the mountains or someplace wide open. I can't seem to escape the feeling of being in an ever-shrinking box where there is less air to breathe and less space to move. It has actually provoked bouts of panic, where I have to overpower that feeling. Then there is the struggle of overcoming the depression that the panic and claustrophobia bring on. It is mentally and physically taxing for me. That I cannot leave for various reasons makes it feel like I'm not only in a box but also chained up inside the box. I exist in this space, but I don't really live. I just wait for the next thing I need to do or the opportunity to see my children or friends.

The struggle to be around people is real. It requires all my strength to be around people. I have to prepare myself mentally and emotionally, but the struggle has seen a significant increase this last year. That I have to be around people frequently makes me want to breakdown and cry. Boy, that sucks! I'm a fairly intimidating guy, from what people tell me, but the thought of having to be around people makes me feel like a little boy afraid of the dark. Do I let it stop me? NO! But I also cannot wait to remove myself from the presence of people. It might just blow your mind to know I spend Sundays and Wednesdays greeting people at my church. But just as soon as church is over, I want to get out of there as soon as possible. I spend Sunday afternoons preparing myself to go back in the evening. The weird thing (as if the rest isn't weird) is that just as soon as I leave the city, I don't feel this way. I feel like dancing in the middle of the street, and I can breathe. I was literally acting a fool in the parking lot of a hotel out in the desert recently. I was pretending to be plane and skipping. I could breathe, I could relax and I was no longer in the box.

I discovered there are only a handful of people that I am at all comfortable around or really willing to engage with. But nearly every comment they make provokes thoughts and feelings of similarity or comradery. So, I end up monopolizing conversations because I have not been around the people that I'm willing to talk to. Then I feel guilty about it later, which promotes my feeling of not wanting to engage with or be around people. It almost feels like a form of Tourette's. It also makes me feel like I am not being a good friend. I will frequently reach out to apologize for manipulating the conversation earlier.

I have also learned that the ability to read and the ability to write are two very different animals. I wrote a couple of short books in 2020. Reading entails deciphering someone else's thoughts, expressions and use of words, while writing is my own thoughts being put down on paper as my brain allows. This can also be very fatiguing. I feel pressure in front of my head if I push myself too far.

I may have covered this previously; when I worked construction, I could tune out background noises, but I can no longer do that now. Background noises are like a dripping faucet now. They wear me down.

Closing Thoughts

Adaptation and modification are now the rules of everyday life. Learning to adapt to this new life and changing activities to fit this new life is their key to daily survival.

Yet, in all this, they are (I am) just grateful to God to be alive. Glad to be taking part in life and their family's life at any level. Grateful to God they are not sitting in a corner drooling on themselves and having their diapers changed by their loved ones. And, you know what, they are not depressed because they have God in their life.

Some final thoughts for you. Try just treating them normal, but with some additional patience and understanding on your part. They know they are broken, and as they try to pick up the pieces to move forward with this new life of theirs, they will push themselves too far. There are times they will pay a big price physically, mentally, and emotionally for pushing the limits, but they have to go through this. In the immortal words of Dirty Harry, "a man's got to know his limitations". Pushing themselves beyond their limit is where they find limitations. When they need your help, try showing kindness instead of condescension.

Chapter 4 - Friends

It seems to me that a redefining of the term "Friend" is needed in our lives. People keep saying they lost their friends after their brain injury, but you could just as easily say after divorce, after graduating, and so on. I would argue that those were not "Friends" in the first place; those were buddies, acquaintances, and family. Folks are mistaken for what our idea of friends is.

God chose our families for us. He lets us choose our friends from those He puts in our path. It's okay to make people earn the right to be in your inner circle of trusted companions.

1) Family are the people God chose for us to have in our lives for an undetermined amount of time.

They come and go, but they will always be related to us regardless of whether we like them. We didn't choose for them to have access to us. Do not think of them as "friend". Although not categorized as friends, you may enjoy spending time with them, and they may be very important to you.

2) We have many acquaintances; they are people we know and publicly socialize with. They will never truly know us or really be a part of our lives. Do not think of them as "friend". However, because they have access to us, they have an opportunity to move up to "buddy". This means that some kind of mutual benefit has been realized and some level of compatibility achieved.

3) We have some buddies, which are the people we hang out with occasionally and do things with personally or in small groups. To some degree, they know us but have not lived up to what should be our

expectations for a friend. Do not think of them as "friend". They have the opportunity to move up to "friend" status once they prove themselves. They may also move back down to "acquaintance" based on their actions.

4) God's willing, we will have a handful of actual friends. They are the people we know we can count on, always. If we call, they will move Heaven and Earth to be there. They know us! They know our quirks; they know our attitude; they know our beliefs; they know we're damaged, and they will be there if we call. They also know that, within our power to do so, we will be there for them when they call. We allow each other to be our own people. We let each other say what's on our minds. We can be brutally honest with each other. We also won't intentionally harm each other, although we may say hard things to each other. Both sides have to allow that without letting it damage the friendship. At this

point, you have to consider what they say to you, even if you don't like it or at first blush, you think they are wrong. Take it in and mull it over later. Be grateful that they cared enough to say something, even when you think they are wrong. That they were willing to upset or anger you shows that they think it's important for you to hear it. Maybe they are correct, and maybe they are not. We all have blind spots. We also have to learn to read our friends to see what they would be comfortable hearing from us. Some people are, by nature or circumstance, fragile.

Make no mistake; it takes work from both parties for someone to become a friend. It takes work to be a friend in the beginning. It will seem less like work in time as the value of the relationship outweighs any effort put forth. If you want good friends, you also have to be a good friend!

Can I also suggest that you cannot be selfish or cheap and a good friend at the same time? Going broke for your friends does no one any good, but you also have to be generous. Find that balance. Offer to do the driving. Offer to go to them. Offer to pick up the tab after a meal. Offer to help when you see a need. Lend an ear or shoulder as needed. If you just listen, you will find out how you can help your friend/s. Also, acknowledge the generosity of your friends and be genuinely grateful, especially for their time. Appreciate every moment you get with your friends and loved ones. No one owes you a thing except your employer if you have lived up to your end of the arrangement.

I have mistaken all of these from time to time. I have also mistaken loyalty for friendship. Loyalty is important, but that cannot be all there is. It will make me try harder and longer to make it a friendship and sustainable, but sometimes it just doesn't work.

Friendships require maintenance. Call your friend, text your friend, or go see your friend, if you can. Just let them know they matter, asking nothing of them. Let them know that they are on your heart and mind. I learned that from my grandpa, who had a list of people he called just to remind them he cared and they mattered to him.

Keep in mind that people will always come and go from our lives for various reasons. Our lives are constantly changing from the moment of our birth until we draw our final breath. They may only have a momentary and temporary purpose for us, so let them go if you come to that conclusion. God may bring them back again someday, if it's meant to be.

Finally, can I suggest that you enter every relationship as though it is someone you plan to keep by your side for the rest of your life? Maybe that way, you will put in a more visible effort, which they will, in turn, also reciprocate.

Chapter 5 - My Thoughts on Depression

Allow me start this off by saying that I am not a doctor, nor do I have any degrees that to support my conclusions. If you are under a doctor's care for depression or think you need a doctor's care, please follow their directions. The following are my thoughts and suggestions. They are not intended to be medical advice.

This last year has provided a significant increase in the bouts of depression I've had to overcome. Something in the way God made me, He gave me the ability to see and understand what depression is, what it does to me, along with the strength to treat it like the enemy it is. Depression is a yoke that harnesses you and makes you its slave. It breaks you down and controls you until it becomes like an addiction. The longer you're in it, the more it feels normal and like it's the place you live. It consumes your personality and your thoughts. It deters you from participating in life so that it can be your only true love. Depression is an evil taskmaster. That is how I treat it.

I treat depression just like I would some person trying to push me around; at some point, I will push back. I refuse to be bullied. I refuse to be mistreated—all the things I will not accept from other people, I won't accept from depression. I refuse to live under the yoke of depression. I choose to be more than what depression would have me be.

Right or wrong, I have always weighed myself on the scales of who and how I think I should be. So, that comes with a lot of self-reflection. I always want to be more today than I was yesterday, although I'm not always successful in that endeavor. But I found that depression wants me stuck in a cycle of dependence on it. It's like the abusive person in a relationship that tries to control you. All I can say is, break free. You deserve more from life than depression. Whatever advice you would give someone else about leaving an abusive relationship, you should use in your struggle against depression.

I must also say that it is my opinion that a non-Christian is at a severe disadvantage when dealing with depression. They don't have God to lean on. If you want to know more about becoming Christian please go to my website akaJoeBrewer.com. My personal testimony is there.